SJÖGREN'S SYNDROME DIET FOR BEGINNERS AND NEWLY DIAGNOSED

Eliminate Symptoms and Embrace a Life Free from Inflammation, with Strong Immunity and Improved Digestive Health

Chris Preston, RDN

ACKNOWLEDGEMENTS

I would like to express my deepest gratitude to everyone who supported me throughout the journey of creating this book. To my family and friends, your unwavering encouragement and patience have been invaluable.

A special thanks to my team, whose expertise and guidance were crucial in developing the dietary plans and recipes shared in this book. Your insights have been a cornerstone of this work.

I am also deeply grateful to my editor, Michael Jones, for your meticulous attention to detail and for helping shape this book into a comprehensive and accessible guide.

To the support groups and communities who shared their experiences and provided feedback, your contributions have enriched this book and made it more relatable for those living with fructose intolerance.

Lastly, to my readers, thank you for embarking on this journey with me. I hope this book provides you with the knowledge and tools to navigate your dietary needs and improve your quality of life.

COPYRIGHT

Copyright © Chris Preston, RDN. All rights reserved.

No part of this publication may be reproduced, distributed, or transmitted in any form or by any means, including photocopying, recording, or other electronic or mechanical methods, without the prior written permission of the publisher, except in the case of brief quotations embodied in critical reviews and certain other noncommercial uses permitted by copyright law.

This book is intended to provide general information about diet and nutrition. It is not intended as a substitute for professional medical advice, diagnosis, or treatment. Always seek the advice of your physician or other qualified health provider with any questions you may have regarding a medical condition.

TABLE OF CONTENTS

PART I

UNDERSTANDING SJÖGREN'S SYNDROME

Sjögren's syndrome is an autoimmune disease that causes your immune system to go haywire and attack healthy cells instead of invading bacteria or viruses. Your white blood cells, which normally protect you from germs, attack the glands that are in charge of making moisture. When that happens, the glands can't produce tears and saliva, so your eyes, mouth, and other parts of your body dry out.

The condition often accompanies other immune system disorders, such as rheumatoid arthritis and lupus. In Sjögren's syndrome, the mucous membranes and moisture-secreting glands of your eyes and mouth are usually affected first — resulting in decreased tears and saliva.

Although you can develop Sjögren's syndrome at any age, most people are older than 40 at the time of diagnosis. The condition is much more common in women. Treatment focuses on relieving symptoms.

Sjögren's syndrome Types

You might hear your doctor talk about a couple of types of Sjögren's disease:

Primary Sjögren's syndrome: This means you have it without any other autoimmune rheumatic disease.

Secondary Sjögren's syndrome: This term is used to describe Sjögren's that occurs along with another autoimmune or rheumatic disease, such as rheumatoid arthritis, scleroderma, or lupus.

How common is Sjögren's syndrome?

Experts estimate that around 2 million people in the U.S. have Sjögren's syndrome.

Symptoms and Diagnosis

Symptoms

Sjögren's syndrome symptoms can vary from person to person. You may have just one or two, or you may have many. By far, the most common Sjögren's syndrome warning signs are:

Dry mouth that may have a chalky feeling or feel like cotton. You might have trouble swallowing or talking. In the long run, this can contribute to cavities or other tooth problems, as well as mouth infections like candidiasis (thrush).

Dry eyes that may burn, itch, or feel gritty. This can lead to light sensitivity or blurred eyesight.

You might have one or both of these issues. You could have other symptoms, too, including:

Dry throat, lips, or skin

Dryness in your nose

A change in taste or smell

Swollen glands in your neck and face

Skin rashes and sensitivity to UV light

Dry cough or shortness of breath

Feeling tired

Trouble concentrating or remembering things

Headache

Dryness in the vagina

Swelling, pain, and stiffness in your joints

Muscle pain or weakness

Heartburn, a sensation of burning that moves from your stomach to your chest

Acid reflux, when your stomach acid flows back into your throat

Numbness or tingling in some parts of your body

Trouble breathing

The pain and fatigue of Sjögren's syndrome may be serious enough to interfere with your daily life.

Diagnosis

Because so many people with Sjögren's also have another autoimmune disease and Sjögren's symptoms sometimes look a lot like some other diseases, like fibromyalgia or chronic fatigue syndrome, it can sometimes be hard for your doctor to give you a diagnosis.

To get clues, your doctor will give you a physical exam and may ask you questions such as:

Do your eyes itch or burn often?

Are you getting a lot of cavities in your teeth?

Does your mouth get dry? How about your lips?

Do you have stiff or painful joints?

Your doctor may ask you to get some blood tests. They will take some blood from your vein and send it to a lab to get checked.

The blood tests measure the levels of the types of blood cells you have and can show if you have germ-fighting proteins (antibodies) that many people with Sjögren's have. They can also measure inflammation in your body and the amount of certain proteins called immunoglobulins that are part of your body's infection-fighting system. High levels of these can be signs that you have the disease.

Your blood tests can also give your doctor an idea of how well your liver is working and show if there might be any issues with it.

Your doctor also may recommend a few tests related to your eyes and mouth:

Schirmer tear test: This measures how dry your eyes are. Your doctor will put a small piece of paper under your lower eyelid to see how much your eye tears up.

Slit lamp: Your doctor uses this magnifying device to get a close look at the surface of your eye.

Dye tests: Your doctor puts drops of dye in your eyes to check for dry spots.

Salivary flow test: This measures the amount of saliva you make over a certain amount of time.

Salivary gland biopsy: Your doctor will take a tiny piece of a salivary gland, usually from your lower lip, for testing. This can tell them if you have a rare condition called lymphocytic infiltrate, which is a buildup of white blood cells that look like bumps.

In some cases, they also may suggest an imaging test:

Sialogram: Your doctor uses this to show how much saliva flows into your mouth. They'll give you a shot of dye in the salivary glands in front of your ears and use a special kind of X-ray to take pictures of its flow.

Salivary scintigraphy: This imaging test is used to track how quickly a tiny amount of a radioactive substance gets to all of your salivary glands. Your doctor will give you a shot of the substance then track its progress over the next hour.

Causes and Risk Factors

What causes Sjögren's syndrome?

Sjögren's syndrome is an autoimmune disease. Autoimmune diseases happen when your immune system mistakenly damages your body instead of protecting it. Experts aren't sure what makes your immune system attack your glands and cause Sjögren's syndrome.

Primary Sjögren's syndrome happens with no known trigger or cause.

Other health conditions trigger secondary Sjögren's syndrome, especially other autoimmune diseases and some viral infections.

Viral infections that can trigger secondary Sjögren's syndrome include:

Hepatitis C.

Cytomegalovirus (CMV).

Epstein-Barr virus.

Human T-lymphotropic virus 1 (HTLV).

COVID-19.

Any autoimmune disease can trigger secondary Sjögren's syndrome. Some autoimmune diseases that are related to Sjögren's syndrome include:

Rheumatoid arthritis.

Psoriatic arthritis.

Lupus

Even though studies have linked Sjögren's syndrome to other conditions, there's no guarantee you'll develop it if you have these conditions. Similarly, Sjögren's syndrome might make you more likely to develop other autoimmune conditions, but that doesn't mean you definitely will.

What are the risk factors for Sjögren's syndrome?

Anyone can develop Sjögren's syndrome, but certain groups of people are more likely to have it:

Women and people assigned female at birth (AFAB): More than 90% of people with Sjögren's syndrome are AFAB. People assigned male at birth (AMAB) can develop it, but it's much less common.

People with other autoimmune diseases: Around half of people with Sjögren's syndrome have at least one other autoimmune condition.

People between the ages of 45 and 55: Children, younger adults and adults older than 55 can have Sjögren's syndrome, but it usually develops in adults in that age range.

People who have a biological relative with Sjögren's syndrome: Around 10% of people with Sjögren's syndrome have a direct relative (a biological parent or sibling) with it, too.

Complications Associated with Sjögren's Syndrome

The most common complications of Sjögren's syndrome involve your eyes and mouth.

Dental cavities: Because saliva helps protect the teeth from the bacteria that cause cavities, you're more prone to developing cavities if your mouth is dry.

Yeast infections: People with Sjögren's syndrome are much more likely to develop oral thrush, a yeast infection in the mouth.

Vision problems: Dry eyes can lead to light sensitivity, blurred vision and corneal damage.

Less common complications might affect:

Lungs, kidneys or liver: Inflammation can cause pneumonia, bronchitis or other problems in your lungs; lead to problems with kidney function; and cause hepatitis or cirrhosis in your liver.

Lymph nodes: A small percentage of people with Sjögren's syndrome develop cancer of the lymph nodes (lymphoma).

Nerves: You might develop numbness, tingling and burning in your hands and feet (peripheral neuropathy).

Treatment

You'll need to take medicines throughout your life to help you manage your symptoms. You can buy some kinds in a drugstore without a prescription, while your doctor may need to prescribe stronger ones if those don't work well enough.

Eye treatments

Drops called "artificial tears" can keep your eyes from drying out. You'll need to use them regularly throughout the day. There are also gels and ointments that you put on your eyes at night. The advantage of these thicker treatments is that they stick to your eye's surface, so you won't need to apply them as often as the drops. But because ointments they affect your vision, you use them while you sleep.

If artificial tears aren't helping, your doctor may prescribe drugs for your dry eyes, including:

Cequa

Lacrisert

Restasis

Lacrisert is a tiny rod-shaped medicine. You put it into your eye with a special applicator, usually once or twice a day. Cequa and Restasis come in drops, which you use twice a day.

Another treatment option for dry eyes is a procedure called punctal occlusion. This is when your doctor puts tiny plugs into your tear ducts to block them up. This keeps tears from draining away too fast, meaning they stay on your eyes longer and help your eyes stay moist.

Mouth treatments

To help your dry mouth, your doctor may prescribe drugs that boost the amount of your saliva, including:

Cevimeline (Evoxac)

Supersaturated calcium phosphate rinse (NeutraSal)

Pilocarpine (Salagen)

Another option is a prescription for artificial saliva to keep your mouth moist. If you get yeast infections in your mouth, your doctor might prescribe antifungal medicine.

Ask your doctor, dentist, or pharmacist about mouthwashes or sprays that can relieve dryness. You might need to try several until you find a product that works for you. Get regular dental checkups, and ask your dentist if a fluoride treatment might help you.

Other Sjögren's syndrome treatments

Other treatments address some of the less common symptoms of Sjögren's. For instance, if you get heartburn or acid reflux, your doctor may give you medicines that curb the amount of acid in your stomach.

You might take over-the-counter or prescription pain relief drugs to ease joint or muscle pain. Earwax remover that you can buy at the drugstore might help with itching ears.

Your doctor may also suggest a disease-modifying antirheumatic drug (DMARD) called hydroxychloroquine (Plaquenil) to treat joint pain. It's a medication that's also used to treat malaria, lupus, and rheumatoid arthritis.

It's rare, but some people with Sjögren's get symptoms throughout the body, including belly pain, fever, rashes, or lung and kidney problems. For those situations, doctors sometimes prescribe prednisone (a steroid) or another DMARD called methotrexate (Rheumatrex, Trexall).

Surgery

A minor procedure to seal the tear ducts that drain tears from your eyes (punctal occlusion) might help relieve your dry eyes. Collagen or silicone plugs are inserted into the ducts to help preserve your tears.

Sjögren's syndrome Home Remedies

There are a lot of steps you can take on your own to help manage your symptoms.

For dry mouth:

Sip water frequently.

Chew gum or suck on candy to stimulate saliva flow and help keep your mouth moist. Be sure they're sugar-free so you don't get cavities.

Stay away from carbonated drinks and from spicy, salty, acidic, and dry foods. They can irritate your mouth.

If swallowing is difficult, stick to moist foods and sip water while you eat. Using liquid to moisten food can also help if you've lost some of our sense of taste.

Brush and floss twice a day to avoid cavities.

Don't use mouthwashes with harsh <u>Ingredients</u> like alcohol.

Oil pulling, in which you swish olive or coconut oil in your mouth for several minutes, may help ease dryness.

Use edible moisturizing oils like coconut oil or vitamin E on dry areas of your mouth or tongue. Lip balm can soothe dry lips.

Avoid smoking and secondhand smoke, both of which make mouth dryness worse.

If you notice any symptoms of thrush, such as white patches in your mouth, pain, or a burning feeling, see your doctor or dentist.

For dry eyes, nose, or skin:

Avoid things that dry out your eyes, like smoky areas, drafty rooms, smoke, dust, and fans.

Don't wear eye shadow or use creams on your eyelids.

When using a computer, take breaks often to give your eyes a rest.

Wear wraparound sunglasses, moisture chamber glasses, or goggles to protect your eyes from drying air.

Before you go to bed and when you wake up, place a warm, wet washcloth over your eyelids for a few minutes to stimulate your oil glands and ease irritation.

Use a humidifier or vaporizer at night to ease dry eyes, nose, and mouth. The ideal humidity rate is

55%-60%, no matter what the temperature. You might consider an heating, ventilation, and air conditioning (HVAC) system with a whole-house humidifier.

Try a nasal saline spray or gel for dry nose.

Use warm water, not hot, when you bathe or shower if you have dry skin. Instead of using a towel after showering, let yourself "drip dry." Your skin will absorb the moisture from the shower.

Apply moisturizer every day.

PART II

THE ROLE OF DIET IN SJÖGREN'S SYNDROME MANAGEMENT

Autoimmune diseases are conditions in which your immune system mistakenly damages healthy cells in your body. Types include rheumatoid arthritis, Sjögren's disease, Crohn's disease, and some thyroid conditions.

Your immune system usually protects you from diseases and infections. When it senses these pathogens, it creates specific cells to target foreign cells.

Usually, your immune system can tell the difference between foreign cells and your cells.

But if you have an autoimmune disease, your immune system mistakes parts of your body, such as your joints or skin, as foreign. It releases proteins called autoantibodies that attack healthy cells.

Some autoimmune diseases target only one organ. Type 1 diabetes damages your pancreas. Other conditions, such as systemic lupus erythematosus, or lupus, can affect your whole body.

Role of Diet in Autoimmune Diseases

Diet plays a significant role in autoimmune diseases because the immune system is affected by food, and two-thirds of the immune system is located in the gut1. Gut dysbiosis, an imbalance in the gut microbiome, has been closely associated with multiple autoimmune diseases, suggesting that maintaining a healthy gut microbiome benefits autoimmune health. A Western diet, high in fat, sugar, and processed foods, is thought to be linked to inflammation, which might set off an immune response. While there is no one accepted definition of an "autoimmune diet," some research suggests that certain foods may benefit people with an autoimmune condition. Eating more plant-based foods is associated with lower levels of inflammation and a more balanced gut immune response, making a plant-based diet a viable option to reduce autoimmune symptoms and potentially improve immune function. The autoimmune protocol, sometimes called an autoimmune diet or AIP diet, is designed to help reduce pain and inflammation that comes with being on the autoimmune spectrum.

How Diet Impacts Sjögren's Syndrome Symptoms

Sjögren's syndrome can affect the diet, leading to malnutrition and weight loss. Dietary changes can improve symptoms and quality of life. Symptoms that impact food intake and quality of life for Sjögren's patients, such as dry mouth, compromised dentition, and reflux, can be significantly improved through dietary modification. Decreased salivary flow (xerostomia) has been shown to impact the dietary choices of Sjögren's sufferers. Individuals who experience severe xerostomia tend to avoid crunchy foods such as raw vegetables, dry or tough foods such as meats and breads, and sticky foods such as peanut butter. Xerostomia can also affect dental health. Saliva contains enzymes that break down sugars in the things we eat, buffers that neutralize acid and minerals to remineralize teeth. In the absence of saliva, sugars stick to the teeth and increase bacterial proliferation and dental decay. Poor oral health in the form of missing or highly diseased teeth can cause patients to choose softer, more carbohydrate-rich foods that are easier to chew. Since symptoms like dry mouth can lead to individuals choosing a limited variety of tolerable foods, it is extremely important to focus on maintaining a healthy diet. This means having a variety of fruits and vegetables, lean meats and/or vegetable proteins, whole grains, healthy fats, and avoiding saturated fat, added sugars, and excess sodium as much as possible. This can often be difficult given the rough textures of vegetables and other nutritious foods.

Several strategies can help improve the palatability of nutritious foods. Increase protein intake by cooking using moist cooking methods like baking in liquid, boiling, and slow cooking or pressure cooking. Incorporate meats into soups or sauces, add Greek yogurt to smoothies or dips, and try seafoods like fish and shellfish as they tend to be softer. Increase vegetable intake by adding a variety of them to soups, stews, and smoothies, cooking them well and consuming them mashed, or juicing them. Other recommendations include increasing omega-3 fatty acid intake by having fatty fish like salmon several times per week and incorporating healthy oils like olive and flaxseed oils.

Nutritional management of Sjögren's symptoms is not well studied, however, there is evidence that in- creased intake of antioxidants like omega-3 fatty acids and vitamin E can have a positive effect on salivary output, dry eye, and inflammation. Omega-3 fatty acids can be found in food sources such as fish like tuna, salmon, and mackerel (consumed raw or canned), nuts like walnuts, peanuts, peanut butter, and oils like canola, flaxseed, and walnut oil. Vitamin E can be found in foods such as sunflower seeds, almonds, almond butter, avocados, spinach, butternut squash, broccoli, olive oil, trout, and shrimp, to name a few.

The Gut Microbiome and Sjögren's Syndrome

Research suggests that the gut microbiome, the collection of microorganisms residing in the gastrointestinal tract, may play a role in autoimmune conditions like Sjögren's syndrome.

Several studies have indicated alterations in the gut microbiota composition in individuals with autoimmune diseases, including Sjögren's syndrome. These alterations can affect the immune system's balance and contribute to the development or progression of autoimmune conditions.

Specifically, dysbiosis, which refers to an imbalance in the gut microbiota composition, has been observed in Sjögren's syndrome patients. Changes in the abundance of certain bacterial species, as well as alterations in microbial diversity, have been reported in individuals with Sjögren's syndrome compared to healthy controls.

Additionally, the gut microbiome is involved in regulating immune responses and inflammation throughout the body. Dysbiosis can lead to increased gut permeability, allowing bacterial components to enter the bloodstream and potentially trigger immune responses, contributing to autoimmune processes.

Furthermore, emerging research suggests that the gut microbiome may influence the function of mucosal immune cells, such as those found in the salivary and lacrimal glands affected by Sjögren's syndrome. This interaction between the gut microbiome and mucosal immunity could potentially influence the development or exacerbation of Sjögren's syndrome.

However, the precise mechanisms underlying the relationship between the gut microbiome and Sjögren's syndrome are still being investigated, and further research is needed to fully understand how microbial dysbiosis contributes to the pathogenesis of this autoimmune disorder. Nevertheless, modulating the gut microbiota through interventions such as probiotics, prebiotics, or dietary changes may offer potential therapeutic avenues for managing Sjögren's syndrome symptoms.

PART III

BUILDING A SJÖGREN'S-FRIENDLY DIET

While there is no one-size-fits-all, there are some simple guidelines which are likely to benefit the majority of people living with Sjögren's. By incorporating these tips into your life, you can get a head-start in managing your symptoms and boosting your overall health and wellness.

1. Opt for Whole, Unprocessed Foods:

These are foods which have undergone minimal or no processing, and therefore retain most of their vitamins and nutrients, which the body needs to repair and heal. Studies show associations between eating minimally processed foods and reduced inflammatory markers. Whole foods are the cornerstone of a healing Sjögren's diet

2. Minimize Highly Processed Foods:

Likewise, steering clear of highly processed foods is a key element of a Sjögren's-friendly diet. Highly processed foods have been shown time and time again to contribute to inflammation. These foods are often loaded with additives, preservatives and added sugars, which can trigger inflammation and worsen Sjögren's symptoms. Opting for whole, unprocessed foods is a healthier choice to support your well-being and help you manage your symptoms.

3. Eat Wild-caught Oily Fish 2-3 Times Per Week

Omega-3 fatty acids found in salmon, mackerel or sardines work to reduce inflammation by inhibiting the production of pro-inflammatory molecules called cytokines and eicosanoids. By modulating the inflammatory response, omega-3 fatty acids can help alleviate symptoms such as dryness, pain, and fatigue associated with Sjögren's. Additionally, omega-3 fatty acids have been shown to support overall immune function and promote healthy cellular membranes, which may further benefit those of you with Sjögren's.

4. Embrace Herbs and Spices:

Herbs and spices can be your culinary allies when you have Sjögren's. These flavorful additions not only enhance the taste of your dishes but can also offer potential anti-inflammatory and antioxidant benefits. Incorporating a variety of herbs and spices into your meals can be a tasty way to support your well-being. So, don't be shy – get creative in the kitchen and explore the world of seasonings to make your meals both delicious and Sjögren's-friendly.

5. Cut Down on Gluten and Dairy (Under Professional Guidance Only):

While there's no general recommendation for dietary restrictions in Sjögren's, most individuals find relief by avoiding gluten and dairy products. However, this should only be done under professional guidance, since cutting gluten and dairy out of your diet can leave you at risk of deficiencies.

6. Stay Hydrated:

This should go without saying! However, many people forget to drink a recommended minimum 2 - 2.5L of water a day. Dehydration can wreak havoc in the body, and this is more so with Sjögren's, where the feelings of dryness are already prevalent. To help your body function optimally, it is vital to stay well-hydrated. Water, unsweetened herbal teas, and clear homemade broths are some great options, so make sure to sip on these throughout the day.

7. Cut Out Alcohol

It's worth considering the role that alcohol has in your diet. Alcohol can have various effects on the body, including dehydration and inflammation, which can exacerbate Sjögren's symptoms, and especially dryness. Many people with Sjögren's find that limiting or eliminating alcohol can lead to improvements in their overall well-being and symptoms.

Foods to Include for Symptom Management

Maintaining a diet rich in foods with anti-inflammatory effects can reduce dryness symptoms and provide relief from other associated conditions. Some foods high in anti-inflammatory benefits include:

leafy green vegetables

nuts

fruits

turmeric

ginger

garlic

fatty fish

olives and olive oil

avocado

whole grains

How you cook your foods can also affect dry mouth symptoms. Here are some additional tips to make your meals more enjoyable:

If you choose to make a sandwich, consider adding vegetables that are high in moisture, such as cucumbers.

Adding sauces to your meals can ease swallowing, but use creamy sauces in moderation to limit fat content.

Try soups and smoothies as alternatives to dry foods.

Drink with your meals to ease swallowing.

Soften your foods with broth.

Tender-cook your meats to prevent them from drying out.

Foods to Avoid or Limit

Pursuing the Sjögren's diet or a similar anti-inflammatory diet means eliminating common trigger foods and allergens.

Some foods to avoid include:

red meat

processed foods

fried foods

dairy

sugars and sweets

alcohol

soda

gluten

refined grains

safflower, corn, and canola oils

Some foods affect people differently. Though these foods can trigger inflammation and worsen Sjögren's syndrome symptoms, some can be eaten in moderation. This specifically applies to some dairy products, such as yogurt and cheese.

If your symptoms begin to worsen after eating specific foods, consider eliminating them from your diet. Also, discuss your symptoms with your doctor to ensure you receive the best treatment.

PART IV

DELICIOUSLY SIMPLE RECIPES
YOU MUST TRY!

SJÖGREN'S-FRIENDLY BREAKFAST RECIPES

Orange & blueberry Bircher

Ingredients

* 70g porridge oats

* 2 tbsp golden linseeds

* zest of ½ an orange

* ¾ of a 175g tub yogurt

* 2 peeled and chopped oranges

* 4handfuls blueberries from a 150g pack

Preparation

- STEP 1

Mix 70g oats and 2 tbsp golden linseeds with the zest of 1 /2 an orange. Pour over 300ml boiling water and leave overnight. The next day, stir in three-quarters of a 175g tub of yogurt, spoon into glasses or bowls, top with 2 peeled and chopped oranges, the remaining yogurt and 4 handfuls blueberries from a 150g pack.

Spicy Moroccan eggs

Ingredients

- 2 tsp rapeseed oil

- 1 large onion, halved and thinly sliced

- 3 garlic cloves, sliced

- 1 tbsp rose harissa

- 1 tsp ground coriander

- 150ml vegetable stock

- 400g can chickpea

- 2 x 400g cans cherry tomatoes

- 2 courgettes, finely diced

- 200g bag baby spinach

- 4 tbsp chopped coriander

- 4 large eggs

<u>Preparation</u>

- STEP 1

Heat the oil in a large, deep frying pan, and fry the onion and garlic for about 8 mins, stirring every now and then, until starting to turn golden. Add the harissa and ground coriander, stir well, then pour in the stock and chickpeas with their liquid. Cover and simmer for 5 mins, then mash about one-third of the chickpeas to thicken the stock a little.

- STEP 2

Tip the tomatoes and courgettes into the pan, and cook gently for 10 mins until the courgettes are tender. Fold in the spinach so that it wilts into the pan.

• STEP 3

Stir in the chopped coriander, then make 4 hollows in the mixture and break in the eggs. Cover and cook for 2 mins, then take off the heat and allow to settle for 2 mins before serving.

Fig, nut & seed bread with ricotta & fruit

Ingredients

• 400ml hot strong black tea

• 100g dried fig, hard stalks removed, thinly sliced

• 140g sultana

- 50g porridge oat

- 200g self-raising wholemeal flour

- 1 tsp baking powder

- 100g mixed nuts (almonds, walnuts, Brazils, hazelnuts), plus 50g for the topping

- 1 tbsp golden linseed

- 1 tbsp sesame seed, plus 2 tsp to sprinkle

- 25g pumpkin seed

- 1 large egg

- 25g ricotta per person

- 1 orange or green apple, thickly sliced, per person

Preparation

- STEP 1

Heat oven to 170C/150C fan/gas 3½. Pour the tea into a large bowl and stir in the figs, sultanas and oats. Set aside to soak.

- STEP 2

Meanwhile, line the base and sides of a 1kg loaf tin with baking parchment. Mix together the flour, baking powder, nuts and seeds. Beat the egg into the cooled fruit mixture, then stir the dry Ingredients into the wet. Pour into the tin, then level the top and scatter with the extra nuts and sesame seeds.

- STEP 3

Bake for 1 hr, then cover the top with foil and bake for 15 mins more until a skewer inserted into the centre of the loaf comes out clean. Remove from the tin to cool, but leave the parchment on until cold. Cut into slices, spread with ricotta and serve with fruit. Will keep in the fridge for 1 month, or freeze in slices.

Staffordshire oatcakes with mushrooms

Ingredients

For the oatcakes

- 85g porridge oats

- 85g plain wholemeal flour

- ½ tsp dried yeast

For the topping

- 4 tsp rapeseed oil, plus a little for frying

- 320g button mushrooms, sliced

- 4 tomatoes, each cut into 8 wedges

- 4 tbsp milled seeds with flax and chia

- 4 tbsp tahini

- A few coriander sprigs, chopped

Preparation

- STEP 1

For the oatcakes, tip the oats and 350ml water into a bowl and blitz with a stick blender until smooth (alternatively you can use a food processor or liquidizer). Stir in the flour and yeast, cover and leave in the fridge overnight, or leave at room temperature for 2-3 hrs until bubbles appear.

- STEP 2

Use kitchen paper to rub ½ tsp oil round a non-stick frying pan, then heat. Ladle in a quarter of the batter and swirl the pan to cover the base (the oatcakes should be a few millimeters thick, like a crêpe). Cook for 2 mins, then turn and cook for 2 mins more until golden. Make four oatcakes in the same way. If you're following our Healthy Diet Plan, chill two for another day. Will keep, covered in the fridge, for two days.

• STEP 3

To make the topping for two oatcakes, heat 2 tsp oil in a non-stick pan, add 160g mushrooms and fry for 2-3 mins, stirring until softened. Stir in 2 tomatoes, then add 2 tbsp ground seeds and cook for 2 mins more. Reheat the oatcakes in a dry frying pan or the microwave if necessary, then spread each one with 1 tbsp tahini, the mushroom mixture and scatter with a little coriander before serving. On the second day, repeat step 3 with the remaining ingredients.

Orange & raspberry granola

<u>Ingredients</u>

• 400g jumbo oats

• juice 2 oranges (150ml), plus zest of 1/2

• 1 tsp ground cinnamon

• 2 tbsp freeze-dried raspberries or strawberries (see tip)

• 25g flaked almonds, toasted

• 25g mixed seeds (such as sunflower, pumpkin, sesame and linseed)

To serve

* 2 large oranges, peeled and segmented

* mint leaves (optional)

Preparation

* STEP 1

Put 200g oats and 500ml water in a food processor and blitz for 1 min. Line a sieve with clean muslin and pour in the oat mixture. Leave to drip through for 5 mins, then twist the ends of the muslin and squeeze well to capture as much of the oat milk as possible – it should be the consistency of single cream. Best chilled at least 1 hr before serving. Can be kept in a sealed or covered jug in the fridge for up to 3 days.

* STEP 2

Heat oven to 200C/180C fan/gas 6 and line a baking tray with baking parchment. Put the orange juice in a medium saucepan and bring to the boil. Boil rapidly for 5 mins or until the liquid has reduced by half, stirring occasionally. Mix the remaining 200g oats with the orange zest and cinnamon. Remove the pan from the heat and stir the oat mixture into the juice. Spread over the lined tray in a thin layer and bake for 10-15 mins or until lightly browned and crisp, turning the oats every few mins. Leave to cool on the tray.

• STEP 3

Once cool, mix the oats with the raspberries, flaked almonds and seeds. Can be kept in a sealed jar for up to one week. To serve, spoon the granola into bowls, pour over the oat milk and top with the orange segments and mint leaves, if you like.

Green fritters

Ingredients

- 140g courgettes, grated

- 3 medium eggs

- 85g broccoli florets, finely chopped

- small pack dill, roughly chopped

- 3 tbsp gluten-free flour or rice flour

- 2 tbsp sunflower oil, for frying

Preparation

- STEP 1

Squeeze the courgettes between your hands to remove any excess moisture, or tip onto a clean tea towel and twist it to squeeze out the moisture.

• STEP 2

Beat the eggs in a bowl, add the broccoli, courgettes and most of the dill, and mix together. Add the flour, mix again and season.

• STEP 3

Heat the oil in a non-stick frying pan. Put a large serving spoon of the mixture in the pan, then add 2 more spoonfuls so you have 3 fritters. Leave for 3-4 mins on a medium heat until golden brown on one side and solid enough for you to flip over, then flip over and leave to go golden on the other side. Repeat to make 3 more fritters (there is no need to add any more oil to the pan after the first batch). Scatter with the remaining dill to serve.

Overnight oats with apricots & yogurt

<u>Ingredients</u>

For the oats

- 200g oats

- 50g chia seeds

- 1 tbsp vanilla extract

- 550ml almond milk, or cow's milk (if non-vegan)

For the apricots

- 1 tsp rapeseed oil

- 320g pack fresh apricots, stoned and quartered

- 400g pot fortified oat or plain bio yogurt

- 4 tsp sunflower seeds

<u>**Preparation**</u>

• STEP 1

Mix the oats and chia in a bowl with the vanilla and almond milk. Cover and chill overnight.

• STEP 2

Heat the oil in a small non-stick pan. Add the apricots in a single layer, then cover the pan and cook over a low heat for 5 mins, until softened. Stir well and cook a few minutes more if needed – they will cook a little more in the residual heat as they cool. Cover and keep chilled until needed.

• STEP 3

The next day, stir the yogurt into the oats and spoon into tumblers, small jars or small bowls. Top with the cooked apricots and sunflower seeds. Will keep covered and chilled for up to four days.

Pancakes for one

<u>Ingredients</u>

- 1 large egg

- 40g plain flour

- ½ tsp baking powder

- 45ml milk (dairy, nut or oat based)

- 1 tsp butter

- ½ tbsp oil

- maple syrup or honey and berries, to serve (optional)

<u>**Preparation**</u>

- STEP 1

Separate the egg, putting the white and yolk in separate bowls. Mix the egg yolk with the flour, baking powder and milk to make a smooth paste.

- STEP 2

Beat the egg white and a pinch of salt with an electric whisk (or by hand) until fluffy and holding its shape. Gently fold the egg white into the yolk mixture. Be extra careful not to knock any of the air out.

- STEP 3

Heat the butter and oil in a non-stick frying pan. Dollop a third of the mixture into the pan and cook on each side for 1-2 mins or until golden brown. Repeat with the remaining mixture to make three pancakes. Drizzle over some maple syrup or honey and serve with berries, if you like.

Dippy eggs with Marmite soldiers

<u>Ingredients</u>

- 2 eggs

- 4 slices wholemeal bread

- a knob of butter

- Marmite

- mixed seeds

<u>**Preparation**</u>

- STEP 1

Bring a pan of water to a simmer. Add 2 eggs, simmer for 2 mins if room temp, 3 mins if fridge-cold, then turn off heat. Cover the pan and leave for 2 mins more.

- STEP 2

Meanwhile, toast 4 slices wholemeal bread and spread thinly with butter, then Marmite. To serve, cut into soldiers and dip into the egg, then a few mixed seeds.

Rye bread with almond butter & pink grapefruit segments

Ingredients

• 4 tbsp almond butter (make your own with the 'goes well with' recipe, right)

• 1 grapefruit (you will need about 100g flesh)

• 2 slices rye bread, toasted (optional)

Preparation

• STEP 1

Toast your rye bread, if you like. Segment the grapefruit and spoon the fruit, along with any juice, into a small bowl.

• STEP 2

Spread the almond butter onto the rye bread, and top with the grapefruit, drizzling any juice over the top.

Creamy yogurt porridge with apricot, ginger & grapefruit topping

<u>Ingredients</u>

For the topping

• 300g can apricot in fruit juice

• 1 tsp finely grated ginger

• 2 pink grapefruits, segmented, any juice reserved

For the porridge

- 9 tbsp (75g) porridge oat

- 550g pot 0% fat probiotic plain yogurt

Preparation

- STEP 1

For the topping: Tip the apricots and juice into a bowl, add ginger. Blitz half the mixture to a purée with a hand blender. Stir in the grapefruit and juice. Can be made ahead and chilled for up to 1 week.

- STEP 2

For the porridge: Tip 200ml water into a small non-stick pan and stir in porridge oats. Cook over a low heat until bubbling and thickened. (To make in a microwave, use a deep container to prevent spillage as the mixture will rise up as it cooks, and cook for 3 mins on High.) Stir in yogurt – or swirl in half and top with the rest. Top with the apricot mix.

Whole-wheat flatbreads with beans & poached egg

Ingredients

- 2 eggs

For the beans

- 500g carton passata

- 2 small onions, quartered

- 1 medjool date, stoned

- 3 tsp smoked paprika

* 1 tsp balsamic vinegar

* 400g can haricot beans, drained

For the flatbreads

* 100g wholewheat flour

* ½ tsp baking powder

* 100g natural yogurt

<u>Preparation</u>

* STEP 1

Tip the passata into a food processor with the onions, date and paprika, and blitz until completely smooth. Heat in a medium pan, cover and simmer for 10 mins, stirring frequently, to make a thick pulpy sauce. Taste to make sure the onion is fully cooked. If not, add a splash of water and cook a little longer. Stir in the vinegar and beans, then remove from the heat.

• STEP 2

To make the flatbreads, tip the flour and baking powder into a bowl, then stir in the yogurt to make a soft dough. Tip out onto a lightly floured surface and lightly knead, fully incorporating any flour left in the bowl. Halve the mixture and flatten each piece to a rough oval, using your hands or a rolling pin, to a thickness of two £1 coins. Cut slashes through the centre of the ovals a couple of times with a sharp knife, being careful not to cut through an edge.

• STEP 3

Heat a large, non-stick pan, add a flatbread and cook for 1 min each side until firm and slightly puffed, then repeat with the other. Meanwhile, heat a large pan of water and poach the eggs to your liking.

• STEP 4

Warm the beans and serve on top of each flatbread with a poached egg and some black pepper.

Seven-cup muesli

Ingredients

• 3 cups oats

• 1 cup mixed nuts including macadamia if possible

• ½ cup sesame seeds

- ½ cup sunflower seeds

- ½ cup raisins

- ½ cup dried cranberries

- 1 cup dried ready-to-eat apricots, chopped

To serve

- soya or semi-skimmed milk

- chopped fresh seasonal fruit, such as pears, banana, pineapple, papya, passion fruit and grapes

Preparation

- STEP 1

Tip the oats into a large airtight container and add the nuts, seeds, raisins and cranberries. Stir in the apricots.

• STEP 2

To serve, spoon a portion into a bowl, pour over the milk and top with chopped fresh fruit.

SJÖGREN'S-FRIENDLY LUNCH RECIPES

Summer pistou

Ingredients

- 1 tbsp rapeseed oil

- 2 leeks, finely sliced

- 1 large courgette, finely diced

- 1l boiling vegetable stock (made from scratch or with reduced-salt bouillon)

- 400g can cannellini or haricot beans, drained

- 200g green beans, chopped

- 3 tomatoes, chopped

* 3 garlic cloves, finely chopped

* small pack basil

* 40g freshly grated parmesan

Preparation

* STEP 1

Heat the oil in a large pan and fry the leeks and courgette for 5 mins to soften. Pour in the stock, add three-quarters of the haricot beans with the green beans, half the tomatoes, and simmer for 5-8 mins until the vegetables are tender.

* STEP 2

Meanwhile, blitz the remaining beans and tomatoes, the garlic and basil in a food processor (or in a bowl with a stick blender) until smooth, then stir in the Parmesan. Stir the sauce into the soup, cook for 1 min, then ladle half into bowls or pour into a flask for a packed lunch. Chill the remainder. Will keep for a couple of days.

Cod puttanesca with spinach & spaghetti

Ingredients

- 100g wholemeal spaghetti

- 1 large onion, sliced

- 1 tbsp rapeseed oil

- 1 red chilli, deseeded and sliced

- 2 garlic cloves, chopped

- 200g cherry tomatoes, halved

- 1 tsp cider vinegar

* 2 tsp capers

* 5 Kalamata olives, halved

* ½ tsp smoked paprika

* 2 skinless cod fillet or loins

* 160g spinach leaves

* small handful chopped parsley, to serve

<u>Preparation</u>

* STEP 1

Boil the spaghetti for 10 mins until al dente, adding the spinach for the last 2 mins. Meanwhile, fry the onion in the oil in a large non-stick frying pan with a lid until tender and turning golden. Stir in the chilli and garlic, then add the tomatoes.

- STEP 2

Add the vinegar, capers, olives and paprika with a ladleful of the pasta water. Put the cod fillets on top, then cover the pan and cook for 5-7 mins until the fish just flakes. Drain the pasta and wilted spinach and pile on to plates, then top with the fish and sauce. Sprinkle over some parsley to serve.

Lentil Bolognese soup

Ingredients

- 2 tbsp rapeseed oil

- 3 onions, finely chopped

- 3 large carrots, finely diced

- 3 celery sticks, finely diced

* 4 garlic cloves, finely chopped

* 500g carton passata

* 1 tbsp vegetable bouillon powder

* 125g red lentils

* 1 tsp smoked paprika

* 4 sprigs fresh thyme

* 125g wholemeal penne

* 50g finely grated vegetarian Italian-style hard cheese

<u>Preparation</u>

* STEP 1

Heat the oil in a large non-stick pan then fry the onions for a few mins until they start to colour.

Add the carrots, celery and garlic then fry for 5 more mins, stirring frequently, until the vegetables start to soften.

• STEP 2

Pour in the passata, bouillon powder and the lentils with 2l boiling water. Add the smoked paprika, thyme and plenty of black pepper then bring to the boil, cover the pan and simmer for 20 mins.

• STEP 3

Tip in the penne then cook for 12-15 mins more until the pasta and lentils are tender, adding a little more water if necessary. Stir through the cheese, then ladle half the soup into bowls or a wide-necked flask if you're taking it as a packed lunch. Cool the remaining soup (remove the thyme sprigs) and keep in the fridge until required. It will keep well for several days. Reheat in a pan, adding a little extra water if the soup has thickened.

Summer egg salad with basil & peas

Ingredients

- 150g new potatoes, thickly sliced

- 160g French beans, trimmed

- 160g frozen peas

- 3 eggs

- 160g romaine lettuce, roughly torn into pieces

For the dressing

- 1 tbsp extra virgin olive oil

- 2 tsp cider vinegar

- ½ tsp English mustard powder

- 2 tbsp chopped mint

- 3 tbsp chopped basil

- 1 garlic clove, finely grated

- 1 tbsp capers

<u>Preparation</u>

- STEP 1

Cook the potatoes in a pan of simmering water for 5 mins. Add the beans and cook 5 mins more, then tip in the peas and cook for 2 mins until all the vegetables are just tender. Meanwhile, boil the eggs in another pan for 8 mins. Drain and run under cold water, then carefully shell and halve.

- STEP 2

Mix all the dressing ingredients together in a large bowl with a good grinding of black pepper, crushing the herbs and capers with the back of a spoon to intensify their flavours.

• STEP 3

Mix the warm vegetables into the dressing to coat, then add the lettuce and toss everything together. Pile onto plates, top with the eggs and grind over some black pepper to serve.

Butter bean curry wraps

<u>Ingredients</u>

• 2 large wholemeal tortilla wraps

• ½ the butter bean curry (recipe below)

• 2 handfuls of mixed salad leaves

* ½ the raita (recipe below)

<u>Preparation</u>

* STEP 1

Warm the wraps following pack instructions, or for a few seconds on each side over the gas flame of the hob to create a slight char.

* STEP 2

Reheat leftover butter bean curry in a pan over a low heat until piping hot (if it's quite wet, allow it to reduce slightly). Spread the curry over the centre of the wraps, then top with the salad and the raita. Roll up tightly and serve straightaway.

Mango salad with avocado and black beans

Ingredients

- 1 lime, zested and juiced

- 1 small mango, stoned, peeled and chopped

- 1 small avocado, stoned, peeled and chopped

- 100g cherry tomatoes, halved

- 1 red chilli, deseeded and chopped

- 1 red onion, chopped

- ½ small pack coriander, chopped

- 400g can black beans, drained and rinsed

Preparation

- STEP 1

Put the lime zest and juice, mango, avocado, tomatoes, chilli and onion in a bowl, stir through the coriander and beans.

Rustic vegetable soup

Ingredients

- 1 tbsp rapeseed oil

- 1 large onion, chopped

- 2 carrots, chopped

- 2 celery sticks, chopped

- 50g dried red lentils

- 1½ 1 boiling vegetable bouillon (we used Marigold)

- 2 tbsp tomato purée

- 1 tbsp chopped fresh thyme

- 1 leek, finely sliced

- 175g bite-sized cauliflower florets

- 1 courgette, chopped

- 3 garlic cloves, finely chopped

- ½ large Savoy cabbage, stalks removed and leaves chopped

- 1 tbsp basil, chopped

Preparation

- STEP 1

Heat the oil in a large pan with a lid. Add the onion, carrots and celery and fry for 10 mins, stirring from time to time until they are starting to colour a little around the edges. Stir in the lentils and cook for 1 min more.

- STEP 2

Pour in the hot bouillon, add the tomato purée and thyme and stir well. Add the leek, cauliflower, courgette, and garlic, bring to the boil, then cover and leave to simmer for 15 mins.

- STEP 3

Add the cabbage and basil and cook for 5 mins more until the veg is just tender. Season with pepper, ladle into bowls and serve. Will keep in the fridge for a couple of days. Freezes well. Thaw, then reheat in a pan until piping hot.

Broccoli and kale green soup

Ingredients

- 500ml stock, made by mixing 1 tbsp bouillon powder and boiling water in a jug

- 1 tbsp sunflower oil

- 2 garlic cloves, sliced

- thumb-sized piece ginger, sliced

- ½ tsp ground coriander

- 3cm/1in piece fresh turmeric root, peeled and grated, or 1/2 tsp ground turmeric

- pinch of pink Himalayan salt

- 200g courgettes, roughly sliced

- 85g broccoli

- 100g kale, chopped

- 1 lime, zested and juiced

- small pack parsley, roughly chopped, reserving a few whole leaves to serve

Preparation

- STEP 1

Put the oil in a deep pan, add the garlic, ginger, coriander, turmeric and salt, fry on a medium heat for 2 mins, then add 3 tbsp water to give a bit more moisture to the spices.

• STEP 2

Add the courgettes, making sure you mix well to coat the slices in all the spices, and continue cooking for 3 mins. Add 400ml stock and leave to simmer for 3 mins.

• STEP 3

Add the broccoli, kale and lime juice with the rest of the stock. Leave to cook again for another 3-4 mins until all the vegetables are soft.

• STEP 4

Take off the heat and add the chopped parsley. Pour everything into a blender and blend on high speed until smooth. It will be a beautiful green with bits of dark speckled through (which is the kale). Garnish with lime zest and parsley.

Spicy fish stew

<u>Ingredients</u>

- 1 tbsp olive oil

- 2 onions, thinly sliced

- 3 spring onions, chopped

- 3 garlic cloves, chopped

- 1 red chilli, seeded and thinly sliced

- few thyme sprigs

- 2 x 400g cans chopped tomatoes

- 400ml vegetable bouillon made with 2 tsp vegetable bouillon powder

- 2 green peppers, seeded and cut into pieces

* 160g brown basmati rice

* 400g can and 210g can red kidney beans, drained

* handful fresh coriander, chopped, plus a few sprigs extra

* handful flat-leaf parsley, chopped

* 550g pack frozen wild salmon, skinned and cut into large pieces

* 1 lime, zested

Preparation

* STEP 1

Heat the oil in a large non-stick pan and fry the onions for 8-10 mins until softened and golden. Add the spring onions, garlic, chilli and thyme. Cook, stirring, for 1 min. Pour in the tomatoes and bouillon, then stir in the peppers. Cover and leave to simmer for 15 mins.

• STEP 2

Meanwhile, cook the rice according to pack instructions. Stir in the beans with the coriander and parsley, then leave to cook gently for another 10 mins until the peppers are tender. Add the salmon and lime zest and cook for 4-5 mins until cooked through.

• STEP 3

Ladle into bowls and scatter with the coriander sprigs.

Salmon salad with sesame dressing

Ingredients

For the salad

- 250g new potatoes, sliced

- 160g French beans, trimmed

- 2 wild salmon fillets

- 80g salad leaves

- 4 small clementines, 3 sliced, 1 juiced

- handful of basil, chopped

- handful of coriander, chopped

For the dressing

- 2 tsp sesame oil

- 2 tsp tamari

- ½ lemon, juiced

- 1 red chilli, deseeded and chopped

- 2 tbsp finely chopped onion (¼ small onion)

Preparation

- STEP 1

Steam the potatoes and beans in a steamer basket set over a pan of boiling water for 8 mins. Arrange the salmon fillets on top and steam for a further 6-8 mins, or until the salmon flakes easily when tested with a fork.

- STEP 2

Meanwhile, mix the dressing Ingredients together along with the clementine juice. If eating straightaway, divide the salad leaves between two plates and top with the warm potatoes and beans and the clementine slices. Arrange the salmon fillets on top, scatter over the herbs and spoon over the dressing. If taking to work, prepare the potatoes, beans and salmon the night before, then pack into a rigid airtight container with the salad leaves kept separate. Put the salad elements together and dress just before eating to prevent the leaves from wilting

Spaghetti puttanesca with red beans & spinach

Ingredients

- 100g wholemeal spaghetti

- 1 large onion, finely chopped

- 1 tbsp rapeseed oil

- 1 red chilli, deseeded and sliced

- 2 garlic cloves, chopped

- 200g cherry tomatoes, halved

- 2 tsp cider vinegar

- 1 tbsp capers

- 5 Kalamata olives, halved

- 1 tsp smoked paprika

- 210g can kidney beans, drained

- 160g spinach leaves

- small handful of chopped parsley

- small handful of basil leaves

Preparation

• STEP 1

Cook the spaghetti in simmering water for 10-12 mins until al dente. Meanwhile, fry the onion in the oil in a large non-stick frying pan with a lid until tender and turning golden. Stir in the chilli, garlic and cherry tomatoes.

• STEP 2

Add the vinegar, capers, olives and paprika with a ladleful of pasta water. Stir in the beans and cook until warmed through.

• STEP 3

Add the spinach to the pasta water to wilt, then drain well. Toss with the tomato and bean mixture and the parsley and basil, then pile onto plates or in shallow bowls to serve.

Avocado & black bean eggs

Ingredients

- 2 tsp rapeseed oil

- 1 red chilli, deseeded and thinly sliced

- 1 large garlic clove, sliced

- 2 large eggs

- 400g can black beans

- ½ x 400g can cherry tomatoes

- ¼ tsp cumin seeds

- 1 small avocado, halved and sliced

- handful fresh, chopped coriander

* 1 lime, cut into wedges

<u>Preparation</u>

* STEP 1

Heat the oil in a large non-stick frying pan. Add the chilli and garlic and cook until softened and starting to colour. Break in the eggs on either side of the pan. Once they start to set, spoon the beans (with their juice) and the tomatoes around the pan and sprinkle over the cumin seeds. You're aiming to warm the beans and tomatoes rather than cook them.

* STEP 2

Remove the pan from the heat and scatter over the avocado and coriander. Squeeze over half of the lime wedges. Serve with the remaining wedges on the side for squeezing over.

Spinach kedgeree with spiced salmon

Ingredients

- 2 tsp rapeseed oil

- 1 large onion, halved and sliced

- thumb-sized piece of ginger, finely chopped

- ½ tsp cumin seeds

- ½ tsp ground cinnamon

- 6-8 cardamom pods, seeds crushed

- 1½ tsp ground turmeric

- 1½ tsp ground coriander

- 1 red chilli, deseeded and sliced

• 1 garlic clove, finely chopped

• 1 large red pepper, deseeded and roughly chopped

• 70g brown basmati rice

• 375ml vegetable stock, made with 2 tsp bouillon powder

• 160g baby spinach leaves, roughly chopped

For the salmon

• 3 tbsp fat-free natural yogurt

• 1 tbsp finely chopped mint or coriander

• 2 skinless wild salmon fillets

• 1 tbsp toasted almonds, to serve

<u>**Preparation**</u>

- STEP 1

Heat the oil in a large frying pan and fry the onion and ginger for 5 mins or until soft. Add the cumin, cinnamon, crushed cardamom seeds, and 1 tsp each of the turmeric and coriander. Cook for 30 secs until fragrant. Add the chilli, garlic, pepper and rice, stir briefly, then pour in the stock. Cover and simmer for 35 mins or until the rice is tender and the stock has been absorbed. If the rice is cooked but some liquid remains, remove the lid and simmer uncovered to allow the liquid to evaporate. Add the spinach, cover and cook for 3 mins to wilt.

- STEP 2

Meanwhile, prepare the salmon. Heat the grill to medium and line a baking sheet with foil. Mix the yogurt with the mint or coriander and the remaining turmeric and ground coriander. Spread the yogurt mixture over the salmon, then transfer to the prepared baking sheet and grill for 8-10 mins until the fish can be flaked easily with a fork. Top the kedgeree with the salmon fillets or flake the fish into it, and scatter over the almonds to serve.

SJÖGREN'S-FRIENDLY DINNER RECIPES

Prawn & harissa spaghetti

Ingredients

- 100g long-stem broccoli, cut into thirds

- 180g dried spaghetti, regular or wholemeal

- 2 tbsp olive oil

- 1 large garlic clove, lightly bashed

- 150g cherry tomatoes, halved

- 150g raw king prawns

- 1 heaped tbsp rose harissa paste

- 1 lemon, finely zested

<u>**Preparation**</u>

- STEP 1

Bring a pan of lightly salted water to the boil. Add the broccoli and boil for 1 min 30 secs, or until tender. Drain and set aside. Cook the spaghetti following pack instructions, then drain, reserving a ladleful of cooking water.

- STEP 2

Heat the oil in a large frying pan, add the garlic clove and fry over a low heat for 2 mins. Remove with a slotted spoon and discard, leaving the flavoured oil.

- STEP 3

Add the tomatoes to the pan and fry over a medium heat for 5 mins, or until beginning to soften and turn juicy. Stir through the prawns and cook for 2 mins, or until turning pink. Add the harissa and lemon zest, stirring to coat.

• STEP 4

Toss the cooked spaghetti and pasta water through the prawns and harissa. Stir through the broccoli, season to taste and serve.

Giant couscous salad with charred veg & tangy pesto

<u>Ingredients</u>

• 2-3 raw beetroot (320g), peeled and chopped

• 3 red onions (320g), cut into wedges

• 2 green or orange peppers, deseeded and cubed

- 1 tbsp olive oil

- 320g cherry tomatoes

- 200g wholewheat giant couscous

For the pesto

- 7g fresh coriander, roughly chopped

- 15g flat-leaf parsley, roughly chopped

- 1 garlic clove

- 1 green chilli, deseeded

- ½ tsp cumin

- 1 tbsp apple cider vinegar

- 1 tbsp olive oil

- 40g pine nuts, lightly toasted

<u>**Preparation**</u>

- STEP 1

Heat the oven to 200C/180C fan/gas 6. In a bowl, toss the beetroot, onions and peppers together with the oil, then spread out on a large roasting tray lined with baking paper and roast for 35 mins. Scatter over the cherry tomatoes, then return to the oven for 10 mins more until the tomatoes have softened and the vegetables are tender.

- STEP 2

Meanwhile, cook the couscous following pack instructions, then rinse and drain. To make the pesto, put the coriander and half the parsley in a bowl with the garlic, chilli, cumin, vinegar, oil and 25g of the pine nuts. Add 2 tbsp water, then blitz with a hand blender until smooth or use a small food processor.

• STEP 3

Toss the roasted veg and chopped parsley through the couscous and pile on the pesto, then scatter with the remaining pine nuts.

Tomato penne with avocado

Ingredients

- 100g wholemeal penne

- 1 tsp rapeseed oil

- 1 large onion, sliced, plus 1 tbsp finely chopped

- 1 orange pepper, deseeded and cut into chunks

- 2 garlic cloves, grated

- 2 tsp mild chilli powder

- 1 tsp ground coriander

- ½ tsp cumin seeds

- 400g can chopped tomatoes

- 196g can sweetcorn in water

- 1 tsp vegetable bouillon powder

- 1 avocado, stoned and chopped

- 1/2 lime, zest and juice

- handful coriander, chopped, plus extra to serve

Preparation

- STEP 1

Cook the pasta in salted water for 10-12 mins until al dente. Meanwhile, heat the oil in a medium pan.

Add the sliced onion and pepper and fry, stirring frequently for 10 mins until golden. Stir in the garlic and spices, then tip in the tomatoes, half a can of water, the corn and bouillon. Cover and simmer for 15 mins.

• STEP 2

Meanwhile, toss the avocado with the lime juice and zest, and the finely chopped onion.

• STEP 3

Drain the penne and toss into the sauce with the coriander. Spoon the pasta into bowls, top with the avocado and scatter over the coriander leaves.

Vegan carbonara

Ingredients

- 360g wholewheat spaghetti

- 85g unsalted cashew nuts

- 2 tsp bouillon powder

- 2 tsp English mustard powder

- 1 tsp olive oil

- 200g baby chestnut mushrooms, halved and thinly sliced

- 3 garlic cloves, 2 finely grated

- 1 tsp smoked paprika

- 2 courgettes (about 320g), peeled then grated

- 4 tsp nutritional yeast flakes, optional

- 320g spinach, half cooked each evening as a side dish

Preparation

- STEP 1

Boil the spaghetti for 10 mins or following pack Preparationuntil al dente, reserving a little of the water. Put the cashews, bouillon and mustard in a bowl, then pour over 350ml boiling water.

- STEP 2

Heat the oil in a large non-stick pan. Add the mushrooms and grated garlic, and stir-fry over a high heat until the mushrooms are cooked and starting to crisp up. Take off the heat, stir in the paprika, then tip onto a plate and set aside.

• STEP 3

Add the grated courgette to the pan and cook, stirring every now and then until softened. Meanwhile, whizz the soaked cashews, whole garlic clove and nutritional yeast flakes, if using, with a hand blender until completely smooth. Tip the mixture into the pan with the courgettes and briefly stir over the heat.

• STEP 4

Add the spaghetti and toss in the cashew and courgette mixture until well coated, then toss through the smoky mushrooms. erve half with half the spinach on the side, and chill the rest for another day. Will keep for three days. Reheat in a covered pan with a dash of water, and cook the remaining spinach to serve on the side.

Noodle salad with sesame dressing

<u>Ingredients</u>

For the dressing

- 1 tbsp sesame oil

- 2 tsp tamari

- 1 lemon, juiced

- 1 red chilli, deseeded and finely chopped

For the salad

- 1 small onion, finely chopped

- 2 wholemeal noodle nests (about 100g)

- 160g sugar snap peas

- 4 small clementines, peeled and chopped

* 160g shredded carrots

* large handful of coriander, chopped

* 50g roasted unsalted cashews

Preparation

* STEP 1

Mix all the dressing ingredients together in a large bowl, then stir in the onion. Meanwhile, cook the noodles in a pan of boiling water for 5 mins, adding the sugar snap peas halfway through the cooking time – the noodles and peas should be just tender. Drain, cool under cold running water and drain again. Snip or cut the noodles into smaller lengths to make them more manageable to eat.

• STEP 2

Tip the noodles and peas into the bowl with the dressing, along with the clementines, carrots, coriander and cashews. Toss to combine, then serve in bowls or pack into rigid airtight containers to take to work.

Meatballs with fennel & balsamic beans & courgette noodles

<u>Ingredients</u>

• 400g lean beef steak mince

• 2 tsp dried oregano

• 1 large egg

• 8 garlic cloves, 1 finely grated, the other sliced

- 1-2 tbsp olive oil

- 1 fennel bulb, finely chopped, fronds reserved

- 2 carrots, finely chopped

- 500g carton passata

- 4 tbsp balsamic vinegar

- 600ml reduced-salt vegetable bouillon

For the courgette noodles

- 1 tsp rapeseed oil

- 1-2 large courgettes, cut into noodles with a julienne peeler or spiralizer

- 350g frozen soya beans, thawed

<u>**Preparation**</u>

- STEP 1

Put the mince, oregano, egg and grated garlic in a bowl and grind in some black pepper. Mix together thoroughly and roll into 16 balls.

- STEP 2

Heat the oil in a large sauté pan over a medium-high heat, add the meatballs and fry, moving them around the pan so that they brown all over – be careful as they're quite delicate and you don't want them to break up. Once brown, remove them from the pan. Reduce the heat slightly and add the fennel, carrots and sliced garlic to the pan and fry, stirring until they soften, about 5 mins.

- STEP 3

Tip in the passata, balsamic vinegar and bouillon, stir well, then return the meatballs to the pan, cover and cook gently for 20-25 mins.

- STEP 4

Meanwhile, heat the 1 tsp of oil in a non-stick pan and stir-fry the courgette with the beans to heat through and soften. Serve with the meatballs and scatter with any fennel fronds.

Cumin-spiced halloumi with corn & tomato slaw

Ingredients

- 1 lime, zested and juiced

- 1 tsp rapeseed oil

- 1 tsp fresh thyme leaves

- ¼ tsp turmeric

- ¼ tsp cumin seeds

- 1 tbsp finely chopped coriander

- 1 garlic clove, finely grated

- 100g halloumi, thinly sliced

For the slaw

* 1 lime, zested and juiced

* 3 tbsp bio yogurt

* 3 tbsp finely chopped coriander

* 1 red chilli, deseeded and chopped

* 160g corn, cut from 2 fresh cobs

* 1 red pepper, deseeded and chopped

* 100g fine green beans, blanched, trimmed and halved

* 200g cherry tomatoes, halved

* 1 red onion, halved and finely sliced

* 320g white cabbage, finely sliced

<u>**Preparation**</u>

- STEP 1

Mix the lime zest and juice with the oil, thyme, turmeric, cumin, coriander and garlic together in a bowl. Add the halloumi and carefully turn it until coated – take care as it breaks easily.

- STEP 2

To make the slaw, mix the lime juice and zest, yogurt, coriander and chilli together, then stir in the corn, red pepper, beans, tomatoes, onion and cabbage.

- STEP 3

Heat a large non-stick frying pan or griddle pan and fry the cheese in batches for 1 min each side. Serve the slaw on plates with the halloumi slices on top. If you're cooking for two people, serve half of the halloumi and slaw and chill the rest for lunch another day.

Stir-fried chicken with broccoli & brown rice

<u>Ingredients</u>

* 200g trimmed broccoli florets (about 6), halved

* 1 chicken breast (approx 180g), diced

* 15g ginger, cut into shreds

* 2 garlic cloves, cut into shreds

* 1 red onion, sliced

* 1 roasted red pepper, from a jar, cut into cubes

* 2 tsp olive oil

- 1 tsp mild chilli powder

- 1 tbsp reduced-salt soy sauce

- 1 tbsp honey

- 250g pack cooked brown rice

<u>Preparation</u>

- STEP 1

Put the kettle on to boil and tip the broccoli into a medium pan ready to go on the heat. Pour the water over the broccoli then boil for 4 mins.

- STEP 2

Heat the olive oil in a non-stick wok and stir-fry the ginger, garlic and onion for 2 mins, add the mild chilli powder and stir briefly. Add the chicken and stir-fry for 2 mins more. Drain the broccoli and reserve the water. Tip the broccoli into the wok with the soy, honey, red pepper and 4 tbsp broccoli water then cook until heated through. Meanwhile, heat the rice following the pack <u>Preparation</u>and serve with the stir-fry.

Chicken & chorizo ragu

<u>Ingredients</u>

• 120g cooking chorizo, chopped

• 1 red onion, chopped

• 2 garlic cloves, grated

• 1 tsp hot smoked paprika

• 80g sundried tomatoes, roughly chopped

• 600g skinless and boneless chicken thighs

- 400g can chopped tomatoes

- 100ml chicken stock

- 1 lemon, juiced

- jacket potatoes, chopped parsley and soured cream, to serve (optional)

<u>Preparation</u>

- STEP 1

Fry the chorizo over a medium heat in a large saucepan or flameproof casserole dish for 5 mins or until it releases its oil and starts to char at the edges. Add the onion and fry for 5 mins more or until soft. Tip in the garlic and cook for 2 mins before stirring in the paprika and sundried tomatoes. Add the chicken thighs and fry for 2 mins each side until they are well coated in the spices and beginning to brown.

• STEP 2

Pour in the chopped tomatoes and stock, and turn the heat down. Cover and cook for 40 mins until the chicken is falling apart and the sauce is thick. Stir the lemon juice through. Serve by piling spoonfuls of the ragu into hot jacket potatoes with parsley sprinkled over and a dollop of soured cream, if you like.

Steaks with goulash sauce & sweet potato fries

Ingredients

• 3 tsp rapeseed oil, plus extra for the steaks

• 250g sweet potatoes, peeled and cut into narrow chips

- 1 tbsp fresh thyme leaves

- 2 small onions, halved and sliced (190g)

- 1 green pepper, deseeded and diced

- 2 garlic cloves, sliced

- 1 tsp smoked paprika

- 85g cherry tomatoes, halved

- 1 tbsp tomato purée

- 1 tsp vegetable bouillon powder

- 2 x 125g fillet steaks, rubbed with a little rapeseed oil

- 200g bag baby spinach, wilted in a pan or the microwave

<u>**Preparation**</u>

- STEP 1

Heat oven to 240C/220C fan/gas 7 and put a wire rack on top of a baking tray. Toss the sweet potatoes and thyme with 2 tsp oil in a bowl, then scatter them over the rack and set aside until ready to cook.

- STEP 2

Heat 1 tsp oil in a non-stick pan, add the onions, cover the pan and leave to cook for 5 mins. Take off the lid and stir – they should be a little charred now. Stir in the green pepper and garlic, cover the pan and cook for 5 mins more. Put the potatoes in the oven and bake for 15 mins.

- STEP 3

While the potatoes are cooking, stir the paprika into the onions and peppers, pour in 150ml water and stir in the cherry tomatoes, tomato purée and bouillon. Cover and simmer for 10 mins.

• STEP 4

Pan-fry the steak in a hot, non-stick pan for 2-3 mins each side depending on their thickness. Rest for 5 mins. Spoon the goulash sauce onto plates and top with the beef. Serve the chips and spinach alongside.

Minty griddled chicken & peach salad

Ingredients

- 1 lime, zested and juiced

- 1 tbsp rapeseed oil

- 2 tbsp mint, finely chopped, plus a few leaves to serve

- 1 garlic clove, finely grated

- 2 skinless chicken breast fillets (300g)

- 160g fine beans, trimmed and halved

- 2 peaches (200g), each cut into 8 thick wedges

- 1 red onion, cut into wedges

- 1 large Little Gem lettuce (165g), roughly shredded

- ½ x 60g pack rocket

- 1 small avocado, stoned and sliced

- 240g cooked new potatoes

<u>Preparation</u>

- STEP 1

Mix the lime zest and juice, oil and mint, then put half in a bowl with the garlic. Thickly slice the chicken at a slight angle, add to the garlic mixture and toss together with plenty of black pepper.

- STEP 2

Cook the beans in a pan of water for 3-4 mins until just tender. Meanwhile, griddle the chicken and onion for a few mins each side until cooked and tender. Transfer to a plate, then quickly griddle the peaches. If you don't have a griddle pan, use a non-stick frying pan with a drop of oil.

• STEP 3

Toss the warm beans and onion in the remaining mint mixture, and pile onto a platter or into individual shallow bowls with the lettuce and rocket. Top with the avocado, peaches and chicken and scatter over the mint. Serve with the potatoes while still warm.

Spinach kedgeree with spiced salmon

<u>Ingredients</u>

• 2 tsp rapeseed oil

• 1 large onion, halved and sliced

- thumb-sized piece of ginger, finely chopped

- ½ tsp cumin seeds

- ½ tsp ground cinnamon

- 6-8 cardamom pods, seeds crushed

- 1½ tsp ground turmeric

- 1½ tsp ground coriander

- 1 red chilli, deseeded and sliced

- 1 garlic clove, finely chopped

- 1 large red pepper, deseeded and roughly chopped

- 70g brown basmati rice

- 375ml vegetable stock, made with 2 tsp bouillon powder

* 160g baby spinach leaves, roughly chopped

For the salmon

* 3 tbsp fat-free natural yogurt

* 1 tbsp finely chopped mint or coriander

* 2 skinless wild salmon fillets

* 1 tbsp toasted almonds, to serve

<u>Preparation</u>

* STEP 1

Heat the oil in a large frying pan and fry the onion and ginger for 5 mins or until soft. Add the cumin, cinnamon, crushed cardamom seeds, and 1 tsp each of the turmeric and coriander. Cook for 30 secs until fragrant. Add the chilli, garlic, pepper and rice, stir briefly, then pour in the stock. Cover and simmer for 35 mins or until the rice is tender and the stock has been absorbed. If the rice is cooked but some liquid remains, remove the lid and simmer uncovered to allow the liquid to evaporate. Add the spinach, cover and cook for 3 mins to wilt.

• STEP 2

Meanwhile, prepare the salmon. Heat the grill to medium and line a baking sheet with foil. Mix the yogurt with the mint or coriander and the remaining turmeric and ground coriander. Spread the yogurt mixture over the salmon, then transfer to the prepared baking sheet and grill for 8-10 mins until the fish can be flaked easily with a fork. Top the kedgeree with the salmon fillets or flake the fish into it, and scatter over the almonds to serve.

SJÖGREN'S-FRIENDLY   SNACKS RECIPES

Weaning recipe: Fish pie bites

Ingredients

- 1 medium baking potato

- 1 small salmon fillet, about 120g

- 1 tbsp frozen sweetcorn and peas, defrosted

- 1 tsp fresh chives, snipped into little strands

- 25g mild cheddar, grated

- ½ small egg, beaten

- oil, for greasing

<u>**Preparation**</u>

• STEP 1

Heat the oven to 200C/ 180 fan/ gas 6. Wrap the potato in foil, place on a baking tray and roast in the oven for 1 hour 15 mins. Wrap the fish in foil, put on the same tray and continue cooking for around 10- 12 mins until opaque and cooked through.

• STEP 2

Once cooked, halve the potato and scoop out the filling. Flake the fish, removing any bones and discarding the skin.

• STEP 3

Grease a baking tray with a little oil. Mash the potato, then mix through the flaked fish, veg, chives, cheese and egg. Allow to cool a little, then take golf-ball sized dollops of mixture and form into little croquette shapes. Arrange on a foil-lined tray and chill in the fridge for 30 mins. If freezing, put the tray in the freezer instead. Once frozen, transfer to a freezer bag and take them out when needed. Thoroughly defrost in the fridge before cooking.

• STEP 4

To cook, heat the oven to 200C/ 180 fan/ gas 6. Arrange as many as you need on a baking tray and cook for around 15 mins or until golden and cooked through. The inside will be very hot so make sure it's sufficiently cooled before serving to your little one.

Chia & almond overnight oats

Ingredients

- 200g jumbo porridge oats

- 50g chia seeds

- 600ml unsweetened almond milk, plus 8 tbsp

- 2 tsp vanilla extract

- 125g punnet raspberries

- 100g almond yogurt

- 250g punnet blueberries

- 20g flaked almonds, toasted

Preparation

- STEP 1

Tip the oats and seeds into a bowl and pour over the milk and vanilla extract. Leave for 5-10 mins for the oats to absorb some of the liquid.

- STEP 2

Reserve 16 raspberries, then add the remainder to the oats and crush them into the mixture. Spoon into four tumblers or sundae dishes, then top with the yogurt and both lots of berries. Cover and chill overnight or until needed. To serve, pour 2 tbsp almond milk over each and scatter with the almonds.

Instant frozen berry yogurt

Ingredients

- 250g frozen mixed berry

- 250g Greek yogurt

- 1tbsp honey or agave syrup

Preparation

- STEP 1

Blend berries, yogurt and honey or agave syrup in a food processor for 20 seconds, until it comes together to a smooth ice-cream texture. Scoop into bowls and serve.

Chia & oat breakfast scones with yogurt and berries

Ingredients

- 2 tsp cold pressed rapeseed oil, plus a little for the ramekins

- 50ml milk

- 1 tbsp lemon juice

- 2 tsp vanilla extract

- 160g plain wholemeal spelt flour

- 2 tbsp chia seeds

- 25g oats

- 2 tsp baking powder

- 2 x 120g pots bio Greek yogurt

- 400g strawberries, hulled and sliced

Preparation

- STEP 1

Heat oven to 200C/180C fan/gas 6 and line the base of 4 x 185ml ramekins with a disc of baking parchment and oil the sides with the rapeseed oil. Measure the milk in a jug and make up to 300ml with water. Stir in the lemon juice, vanilla and the 2 tsp oil. Mix the flour, seeds and oats then blitz in a food processor to make the mix as fine as you can. Stir in the baking powder.

- STEP 2

Pour in the liquid, then stir in with the blade of a knife until you have a very wet batter like dough. Spoon evenly into the ramekins then bake on a baking sheet for 20 mins until risen – they don't have to be golden but should feel firm. Cool for a few mins then run a knife round the inside of the ramekins to loosen the scones then carefully ease out. The scones can be eaten immediately or cooled and stored for later.

Polenta bruschetta with tapenade

Ingredients

• 700ml vegetable stock (Marigold Swiss vegetable bouillon is gluten and dairy-free)

• 140g instant polenta

• 2 tbsp chopped fresh basil

• 2 tbsp olive oil

• 9 tsp (about half a 190g jar) olive tapenade

- 9 SunBlush or semi-dried tomatoes, halved

- 100g mixed salad leaves

<u>Preparation</u>

- STEP 1

Bring the stock to the boil in a saucepan, then reduce to a simmer. Stirring continuously, pour in the polenta in a steady steam and cook for 5 mins until thickened. Stir in the basil and season with black pepper and salt, if you like. Spread on an oiled shallow tin measuring 24 x 18cm. Leave to set for 1 hr.

- STEP 2

Cut the polenta into 9 rectangles, each 8 x 6cm, then cut in half diagonally to make triangle shapes. Heat a griddle until hot, brush each triangle with oil and grill for 4-5 mins each side, until crisp and golden.

• STEP 3

Top each triangle with 1/2 tsp tapenade and half a tomato. Serve warm on salad leaves.

Quinoa porridge

Ingredients

For the porridge (to serve 4)

- 175g quinoa

- ½ vanilla pod, split and seeds scraped out, or 0.5 tsp vanilla extract

- 15g creamed coconut

- 4 tbsp chia seeds

- 125g coconut yogurt

For the topping (to serve 2)

- 125g pot coconut yogurt

- 280g mixed summer berries, such as strawberries, raspberries and blueberries

• 2 tbsp flaked almonds (optional)

Preparation

• STEP 1

Activate the quinoa by soaking overnight in cold water. The next day, drain and rinse the quinoa through a fine sieve (the grains are so small that they will wash through a coarse one).

• STEP 2

Tip the quinoa into a pan and add the vanilla, creamed coconut and 600ml water. Cover the pan and simmer for 20 mins. Stir in the chia with another 300ml water and cook gently for 3 mins more. Stir in the pot of coconut yogurt. Spoon half the porridge into a bowl for another day. Will keep for 2 days covered in the fridge. Serve the remaining porridge topped with another pot of yogurt, the berries and almonds, if you like.

• STEP 3

To have the porridge another day, tip into a pan and reheat gently, with milk or water. Top with fruit - for instance, orange slices and pomegranate seeds.

Tuna Niçoise protein pot

Ingredients

• 1 large egg

• 80g green beans

• 1 tomato, amber or red, quartered

- 120g can tuna in spring water

- 1½ -2 tbsp French dressing

Preparation

* STEP 1

Boil the egg for 8-10 mins depending on if you want a soft or hard yolk, then at the same time steam the green beans for 6 mins above the pan until tender. Cool the egg and beans under running water then carefully shell and quarter the egg. Leave to cool.

* STEP 2

Tip the beans into a large packed lunch pot. Top with the tomato, tuna and quartered egg and spoon on the French dressing. Seal until ready to eat.

Homemade vegan bagels

Ingredients

- 7g sachet dried yeast

- 4 tbsp sugar

- 2 tsp salt

- 450g bread flour

- poppy, fennel and/or sesame seeds to sprinkle on top (optional)

Preparation

- STEP 1

Tip the yeast and 1 tbsp sugar into a large bowl, and pour over 100ml warm water. Leave for 10 mins until the mixture becomes frothy.

- STEP 2

Pour 200ml warm water into the bowl, then stir in the salt and half the flour. Keep adding the remaining flour (you may not have to use it all) and mixing with your hands until you have a soft but not sticky dough. Then knead for 10 mins until the dough feels smooth and elastic. Shape into a ball and put in a clean, lightly oiled bowl. Cover loosely and leave in a warm place until doubled in size, about 1hr.

- STEP 3

Heat the oven to 220C/200C fan/gas 7. On a lightly floured surface, divide the dough into 10 pieces, each about 85g. Shape each piece into a flattish ball, then take a wooden spoon and use the handle to make a hole in the middle of each ball. Slip the spoon into the hole, then twirl the bagel around the spoon to make a hole about 3cm wide. Cover the bagel loosely while you shape the remaining dough.

• STEP 4

Meanwhile, bring a large pan of water to the boil and tip in the remaining sugar. Slip the bagels into the boiling water – no more than four at a time. Cook for 1-2 mins, turning over in the water until the bagels have puffed slightly and a skin has formed. Remove with a slotted spoon and drain away any excess water. Sprinkle over your choice of topping and place on a baking tray lined with parchment. Bake in the oven for 25 mins until browned and crisp – the bases should sound hollow when tapped. Leave to cool on a wire rack, then serve with your favourite filling.

Puff pastry pizzas

<u>Ingredients</u>

- 320g sheet ready-rolled light puff pastry

- 6 tbsp tomato purée

- 1 tbsp tomato ketchup

- 1 tsp dried oregano

- 75g mozzarella or cheddar

For the topping

- sweetcorn, olives, peppers, red onion, cherry tomatoes, spinach, basil

<u>**Preparation**</u>

• STEP 1

Heat the oven to 200C/180C fan/gas 6, or if using an air-fryer, heat it to 180C for 4 mins. Unroll the pastry, cut into six squares and arrange over two baking trays lined with baking parchment. Use a cutlery knife to score a 1cm border around the edge of each pastry square. Bake in the oven for 15 mins, until puffed up but not cooked through. Or, if using an air-fryer, bake the batch for 8 mins. You might need to do this in two batches.

• STEP 2

While the pastry cooks, make the sauce and prepare your toppings. Mix the tomato purée, tomato ketchup, oregano and 1 tbsp water. Grate the cheese and chop any veg or herbs you want to put on top into small pieces. Set aside.

• STEP 3

Remove the pastry from the oven or air-fryer and squash down the middles with the back of a spoon. Divide the sauce between the pastry squares and spread it out to the puffed-up edges. Sprinkle with the cheese, then add your toppings. Bake for another 5-8 mins in the oven or 5 mins in the air-fryer and serve.

Sweetcorn fritters

<u>Ingredients</u>

- 150g self-raising flour

- 1 tsp baking powder

- 1 tsp smoked paprika

- 160ml whole milk

- 1 egg

- 550g sweetcorn

- 2 spring onions, chopped, plus a little extra cut into thin strips to serve (optional)

- 10g sliced chives

- handful of parsley, chopped

- rapeseed oil, for frying

Preparation

- STEP 1

Mix the flour, baking powder, paprika and milk together in a large bowl. Mix in the egg, followed by the sweetcorn, chopped spring onions, chives, parsley, 1 tsp salt and some freshly ground black pepper.

- STEP 2

Heat a 1cm depth of oil in a frying pan over a medium heat until a small amount of the fritter mixture sizzles when dropped in. For larger fritters, drop 2 heaped tablespoons of the mixture into the pan at a time in a clockwise direction (this will help you remember the order they were added to the pan, so you can flip them at the right stage). For smaller fritters, do the same, but with 1 heaped tablespoon of mixture at a time.

• STEP 3

After 2 mins, flip the fritters over in the same order they were added to the pan. Cook for another 2 mins, continuing to turn every now and then to ensure both sides are evenly golden brown. When ready, the fritters should be darker brown with crispy pieces of corn at the edges – be careful, as some of the kernels may burst during the cooking process. Remove to a wire rack and pat away any excess oil using kitchen paper. Serve straightaway with a few strips of spring onion scattered over, if you like.

Cheese-stuffed garlic dough balls with a tomato sauce dip

Ingredients

- 50g butter, cubed

- 300g strong white bread flour

- 7g sachet fast-action dried yeast

- 1 tbsp caster sugar

- 200g block mozzarella, cut into 1.5cm cubes

- 65g gruyère, coarsely grated (optional)

For the garlic butter

- 100g butter

- 2 garlic cloves, crushed

• 1 rosemary sprig, leaves picked and finely chopped

For the tomato sauce dip

• 1 tbsp olive oil, plus extra for the bowl and baking sheet

• 1 garlic clove, sliced

• 250g passata

• 1 tsp red wine vinegar

• 1 tsp caster sugar

• pinch of chilli flakes

• ½ small bunch of basil, torn, plus extra to serve

<u>Preparation</u>

- STEP 1

Heat 175ml water in a saucepan until steaming, then add the butter. Remove from the heat and leave to cool until the mixture is just warm (it should not be hot). Combine the flour, yeast, sugar and 1 tsp salt in a large bowl or stand mixer. Add the cooled butter mixture, and mix to a soft dough using a wooden spoon or the mixer. Knead for 10 mins by hand (or 5 mins using a mixer) until the dough feels bouncy and smooth. Transfer to an oiled bowl and cover with a clean tea towel. Leave somewhere warm to rise for 1½-2 hrs, or until doubled in size. Alternatively, leave to prove in the fridge overnight.

- STEP 2

Oil and line a baking sheet with baking parchment. Knock the air out of the dough, then knead again for several minutes. Flatten a small piece of dough (about 20g) into a disc, and put a cube of the mozzarella and a pinch of the gruyère into the middle of the disc. Enclose the cheeses with the dough, then roll into a ball. Transfer to the prepared baking sheet. Repeat with the remaining cheese and dough, placing the dough balls ½cm apart on the baking sheet – they should be just touching after proving. Cover with a clean tea towel and leave somewhere warm to rise for 30 mins.

• STEP 3

Meanwhile, make the garlic butter. Melt the butter in a small pan over a low heat, then stir in the garlic and rosemary. Remove from the heat and set aside until needed. Heat the oven to 180C/160C fan/gas

4. Brush the risen dough balls with the garlic butter, then bake for 25-30 mins until the dough balls are cooked through and the middles are oozing.

• STEP 4

While the dough balls are baking, make the tomato sauce dip. Heat the oil in a saucepan and fry the garlic for 30 seconds. Tip in the passata, vinegar, sugar and chilli flakes, and simmer for 10 mins until thickened. Season to taste and stir in the basil. Brush the warm dough balls with any remaining garlic butter, then serve with the tomato sauce dip on the side for dunking.

Easy plum jam

<u>**Ingredients**</u>

- 2kg plums, stoned and roughly chopped

- 2kg white granulated sugar

- 2 tsp ground cinnamon

- 1 tbsp lemon juice

- 3 cinnamon sticks (optional)

- knob of butter

<u>**Preparation**</u>

- STEP 1

Sterilise the jars and any other equipment before you start (see tip). Put a couple of saucers in the freezer, as you'll need these for testing whether the jam is ready later (or use a sugar thermometer). Put the plums in a preserving pan and add 200ml water. Bring to a simmer, and cook for about 10 mins until the plums are tender but not falling apart. Add the sugar, ground cinnamon and lemon juice, then let the sugar dissolve slowly, without boiling. This will take about 10 mins.

• STEP 2

Increase the heat and bring the jam to a full rolling boil. After about 5 mins, spoon a little jam onto a cold saucer. Wait a few seconds, then push the jam with your fingertip. If it wrinkles, the jam is ready. If not, cook for a few mins more and test again, with another cold saucer. If you have a sugar thermometer, it will read 105C when ready.

- STEP 3

Take the jam off the heat and add the cinnamon sticks (if using) and the knob of butter. The cinnamon will look pretty in the jars and the butter will disperse any scum. Let the jam cool for 15 mins, which will prevent the lumps of fruit sinking to the bottom of the jars. Ladle into hot jars, seal and leave to cool. Will keep for 1 year in a cool, dark place. Chill once opened.

Caramelised mushroom tartlets

Ingredients

- 2 tbsp olive oil

- 1 onion, chopped

* 1 tbsp golden caster sugar

* 250g chestnut mushrooms, cleaned and thinly sliced

* 1 garlic clove, crushed

* 3-4 tbsp thyme leaves, finely chopped

* butter, for spreading

* 12 slices of thin sliced white sandwich bread

* 100g grated gruyère or cheddar, for sprinkling

Preparation

* STEP 1

Heat the oil in a generous frying pan, add the onion and fry over moderate heat for about 7 mins until soft and golden. Stir in the sugar and seasoning, turn up the heat and add the mushrooms. Sizzle for 5 mins until you have driven off any moisture and the mushrooms are golden. Stir in the garlic for a few further mins, until fragrant, then turn off the heat and stir in most of the thyme (save some for sprinkling). The mushroom mix can be chilled at this point.

• STEP 2

To make the tartlet bases, cut 7-8cm circles out of the bread using a cookie cutter or glass. Butter one side and stick buttered-side down into a 12-hole tartlet tin. Freeze any leftovers to make breadcrumbs.

• STEP 3

When ready to bake, heat oven to 220C/200 fan/gas 7. Divide the mushroom mixture between the tartlets and top with a sprinkle of cheese. Don't be too tidy about this – any cheese on the tin will form a lacy edge to the tartlets. Bake for 10-15 mins until golden and bubbling. Sprinkle over the reserved herbs and serve.

Ricotta and basil pizza

Ingredients

- 1 onion, finely chopped

- 2 yellow peppers, roughly chopped

- 1 tsp olive oil

- 2 x 400g/14oz cans chopped tomatoes

- 500g bag mixed grain or granary bread mix

- plain flour, for dusting

* 10 cherry tomatoes, halved or whole

* 250g tub ricotta

* a few basil leaves, to serve

Instructions

* STEP 1

Heat oven to 220C/fan 200C/gas 6. Soften the onion and peppers in the oil in a large pan for a few mins. Pour in the tomatoes, season, then simmer for 10 mins.

* STEP 2

Meanwhile, make up the bread mix according to pack instructions, then bring the dough together and knead a couple of times. Flour a large baking sheet and roll out the dough into a rectangle roughly 25 x 35cm. Bake for 5 mins on a shelf at the top of the oven until firm.

• STEP 3

Remove from the oven, spread with the sauce, add the cherry tomatoes, then dollop over spoonfuls of the ricotta. Bake for 10 mins more until the base is golden and crisp. Scatter with basil and serve straight away with a green salad.

SJÖGREN'S-FRIENDLY RECIPES

Corn & split pea chowder

<u>Ingredients</u>

200g dried yellow split peas

3 celery sticks (about 160g), sliced

1 thyme sprig, plus 1 tbsp thyme leaves

2 onions (350g), halved and sliced

1 tbsp rapeseed oil

50g ginger, finely grated

2 red chillies, deseeded and sliced

3 garlic cloves, chopped

1 large green pepper, chopped into small pieces

1 potato (about 215g), unpeeled, cut into 1-2cm pieces

2 tbsp vegetable bouillon powder

320g frozen sweetcorn

150g coconut yogurt

<u>Preparation</u>

STEP 1

Tip the split peas, celery and thyme sprig into a medium pan with 1 litre of boiling water, bring back to the boil and simmer, covered, for 25 mins.

STEP 2

Meanwhile, fry the onion in the oil in a large pan for 10 mins. Stir in the ginger, chilli and garlic. Tip in the pepper and potato, and pour in ½ litre boiling water with the bouillon and remaining thyme. Tip in the split pea mixture and corn, bring to the boil, then cover and simmer for 30-35 mins until the veg is tender.

STEP 3

Remove the thyme sprig. Take out a third of the veg, then purée the rest in the pan with a hand blender (or use a potato masher). Return the veg to the pan with the yogurt, and stir well.

Broccoli and kale green soup

Ingredients

500ml stock, made by mixing 1 tbsp bouillon powder and boiling water in a jug

1 tbsp sunflower oil

2 garlic cloves, sliced

thumb-sized piece ginger, sliced

½ tsp ground coriander

3cm/1in piece fresh turmeric root, peeled and grated, or 1/2 tsp ground turmeric

pinch of pink Himalayan salt

200g courgettes, roughly sliced

85g broccoli

100g kale, chopped

1 lime, zested and juiced

small pack parsley, roughly chopped, reserving a few whole leaves to serve

<u>**Preparation**</u>

STEP 1

Put the oil in a deep pan, add the garlic, ginger,
coriander, turmeric and salt, fry on a medium heat
for 2 mins, then add 3 tbsp water to give a bit more
moisture to the spices.

STEP 2

Add the courgettes, making sure you mix well to
coat the slices in all the spices, and continue
cooking for 3 mins. Add 400ml stock and leave to
simmer for 3 mins.

STEP 3

Add the broccoli, kale and lime juice with the rest
of the stock. Leave to cook again for another 3-4
mins until all the vegetables are soft.

STEP 4

Take off the heat and add the chopped parsley. Pour everything into a blender and blend on high speed until smooth. It will be a beautiful green with bits of dark speckled through (which is the kale). Garnish with lime zest and parsley.

Fresh tomato soup with cheesy cornbread

<u>Ingredients</u>

For the bread

40g wholemeal self-raising flour

85g ground polenta

1 tsp baking powder

40g mature cheddar, finely grated

1 tsp smoked paprika

3 spring onions (35g), finely sliced

1 green chilli, deseeded, finely sliced

1 large egg

125ml milk

For the soup

2 tsp rapeseed oil

3-5 sticks celery (165g), finely chopped

2 onions, chopped

4 carrots (320g), diced

325g floury potatoes, grated

500g tomatoes, chopped

4 tsp vegetable bouillon powder made up to 1 1/2 litre with boiling water

3 tbsp tomato purée

2 large garlic cloves, finely grated

flat-leaf parsley, chopped, to serve

Preparation

STEP 1

First, make the bread. Heat oven to 200C/180C fan/gas 6 and line the base of a non-stick 500g loaf tin with baking parchment. Tip the flour, polenta and baking powder into a bowl with half the cheese, the paprika, onions and chilli, then toss together. Add the egg and milk and mix well. Turn out into the tin and top with the remaining cheese. Bake for 20-25 mins until golden and a skewer inserted into the centre comes out clean.

STEP 2

To make the soup, heat the oil in a large pan and fry the celery, onion and carrots for 10 mins until softened. Add the potatoes, tomatoes, bouillon, tomato purée and garlic, then stir well. Cover with a lid and cook for 20 mins.

STEP 3

Remove from the heat and blitz until smooth with a hand blender.

Summer pistou

Ingredients

1 tbsp rapeseed oil

2 leeks, finely sliced

1 large courgette, finely diced

1l boiling vegetable stock (made from scratch or with reduced-salt bouillon)

400g can cannellini or haricot beans, drained

200g green beans, chopped

3 tomatoes, chopped

3 garlic cloves, finely chopped

small pack basil

40g freshly grated parmesan

Preparation

STEP 1

Heat the oil in a large pan and fry the leeks and courgette for 5 mins to soften. Pour in the stock, add three-quarters of the haricot beans with the green beans, half the tomatoes, and simmer for 5-8 mins until the vegetables are tender.

STEP 2

Meanwhile, blitz the remaining beans and tomatoes, the garlic and basil in a food processor (or in a bowl with a stick blender) until smooth, then stir in the Parmesan. Stir the sauce into the soup, cook for 1 min, then ladle half into bowls or pour into a flask for a packed lunch. Chill the remainder. Will keep for a couple of days.

Spinach soup

<u>**Ingredients**</u>

25g butter

1 bunch spring onions, chopped

1 leek (about 120g), sliced

2 small sticks celery (about 85g), sliced

1 small potato (about 200g) , peeled and diced

½ tsp ground black pepper

1l stock (made with two chicken or vegetable stock cubes)

2 x 200-235g bags spinach

150g half-fat crème fraîche

Preparation

STEP 1

Heat the butter in a large saucepan. Add the spring onions, leek, celery and potato. Stir and put on the lid. Sweat for 10 minutes, stirring a couple of times.

STEP 2

Pour in the stock and cook for 10 – 15 minutes until the potato is soft.

STEP 3

Add the spinach and cook for a couple of minutes until wilted. Use a hand blender to blitz to a smooth soup.

STEP 4

Stir in the crème fraîche. Reheat and serve.

Red lentil soup

Ingredients

1 white onion, finely sliced

2 tsp olive oil

3 garlic cloves, sliced

2 carrots, scrubbed and diced

85g red lentils

1 vegetable stock cube, crumbled

generous sprigs parsley, chopped (about 2 tbsp) plus a few extra leaves

<u>**Preparation**</u>

STEP 1

Put the kettle on to boil while you finely slice the onion. Heat the oil in a medium pan, add the onion and fry for 2 mins while you slice the garlic and dice the carrots. Add them to the pan, and cook briefly over the heat.

STEP 2

Pour in 1 litre of the boiling water from the kettle, stir in the lentils and stock cube, then cover the pan and cook over a medium heat for 15 mins until the lentils are tender. Take off the heat and stir in the parsley. Ladle into bowls, and scatter with extra parsley leaves, if you like.

Courgette, pea & pesto soup

Ingredients

1 tbsp olive oil

1 garlic clove, sliced

500g courgettes, quartered lengthways and chopped

200g frozen peas

400g can cannellini beans, drained and rinsed

1l hot vegetable stock

2 tbsp basil pesto, or vegetarian alternative

Preparation

STEP 1

Heat the oil in a large saucepan. Cook the garlic for a few seconds, then add the courgettes and cook for 3 mins until they start to soften. Stir in the peas and cannellini beans, pour on the hot stock and cook for a further 3 mins.

STEP 2

Stir the pesto through the soup with some seasoning, then ladle into bowls and serve with crusty brown bread, if you like. Or pop in a flask to take to work.

Broccoli & stilton soup

<u>Ingredients</u>

2 tbsp rapeseed oil

1 onion, finely chopped

1 stick celery, sliced

1 leek, sliced

1 medium potato, diced

1 knob butter

1l low salt or homemade chicken or vegetable stock

1 head broccoli, roughly chopped

140g stilton, or other blue cheese, crumbled

Preparation

STEP 1

Heat 2 tbsp rapeseed oil in a large saucepan and then add 1 finely chopped onion. Cook on a medium heat until soft. Add a splash of water if the onion starts to catch.

STEP 2

Add 1 sliced celery stick, 1 sliced leek, 1 diced medium potato and a knob of butter. Stir until melted, then cover with a lid. Allow to sweat for 5 minutes then remove the lid.

STEP 3

Pour in 1l of chicken or vegetable stock and add any chunky bits of stalk from 1 head of broccoli. Cook for 10-15 minutes until all the vegetables are soft.

STEP 4

Add the rest of the roughly chopped broccoli and cook for a further 5 minutes.

STEP 5

Carefully transfer to a blender and blitz until smooth.

STEP 6

Stir in 140g crumbled stilton, allowing a few lumps to remain. Season with black pepper and serve.

Chicken & sweetcorn soup

<u>Ingredients</u>

1 chicken carcass

4 thin slices fresh ginger, plus 1 tbsp finely grated

2 onions, quartered

3 garlic cloves, finely grated

2 tsp apple cider vinegar

325g can sweetcorn

3 spring onions, whites thinly sliced, greens sliced
at an angle

100g cooked chicken, shredded

2 tsp tamari

2 eggs, beaten

few drops sesame oil, to serve (optional)

Preparation

STEP 1

Boil a large kettle of water. Break the carcass into a big non-stick pan and add the ginger slices, onion and two-thirds of the garlic. Cook, stirring, for about 2 mins – the meat will stick to the base of the pan, but this will add to the flavour. Pour in 1.5 litres of boiling water, stir in the vinegar, then cover and simmer for 2 hrs.

STEP 2

Put a large sieve over a bowl and pour through the contents of the pan. Measure the liquid in the bowl – you want around 450ml. If you have too much, return to the pan and boil with the lid off to reduce it. Transfer the onion from the sieve to a bowl with three-quarters of the sweetcorn. Blitz until smooth with a hand blender.

STEP 3

Return the broth to the pan, and tip in the puréed corn, remaining sweetcorn and garlic, the grated ginger, the whites of the spring onions and the chicken. Simmer for 5 mins, then stir in the tamari. Turn off the heat, and quickly drizzle in the egg, stirring a little to create egg threads. Season with pepper, then ladle into the bowls. Top with the spring onion greens and a few drops of sesame oil, if using.

Moroccan spiced cauliflower & almond soup

Ingredients

1 large cauliflower

2 tbsp olive oil

½ tsp each ground cinnamon, cumin and coriander

2 tbsp harissa paste, plus extra drizzle

1l hot vegetable or chicken stock

50g toasted flaked almond, plus extra to serve

Preparation

STEP 1

Cut the cauliflower into small florets. Fry olive oil, ground cinnamon, cumin and coriander and harissa paste for 2 mins in a large pan. Add the cauliflower, stock and almonds. Cover and cook for 20 mins until the cauliflower is tender. Blend soup until smooth, then serve with an extra drizzle of harissa and a sprinkle of toasted almonds.

Leek, fennel & potato soup with cashel blue cheese

<u>Ingredients</u>

2 heads fennel

3 large leeks, trimmed, washed and finely sliced

60g butter

1 large potato, peeled and diced

900ml chicken stock or water

1 garlic clove, sliced

100ml double cream

50g walnuts, toasted

75g Cashel Blue cheese, crumbled

<u>Preparation</u>

STEP 1

Quarter the fennel and discard the tough outer leaves and the hard core from each piece. Slice the rest of the flesh, including any little fronds.

STEP 2

Heat the butter in a saucepan and add the fennel, leeks and potato. Cook over a medium heat for about 5 mins, turning the vegetables over in the butter. The vegetables shouldn't colour. Add a splash of water, cover the pan and cook the vegetables for 20 mins, stirring every so often. Add the stock or water and garlic, season, bring to the boil, then turn the heat down low and cover the pan with a lid or foil.

STEP 3

Cook for about 10-15 mins, until everything is completely tender. Stir in the cream and leave to cool. Purée in a blender until completely smooth. Check the seasoning and return the mixture to the saucepan – you can reheat it quickly just before serving. Ladle into bowls and scatter each one with the walnuts and cheese.

Smoky tomato, chipotle & charred corn soup

Ingredients

1 tbsp rapeseed oil

1 onion, finely chopped

2 garlic cloves, chopped

2 tsp ground coriander

small bunch of coriander, stalks chopped and leaves left whole

400g can chopped tomatoes

600ml vegetable stock

1-1½ tbsp chipotle chilli paste

2 corn on the cobs

50g feta, crumbled

4 tbsp fat-free Greek yogurt

<u>Preparation</u>

STEP 1

Heat the oil in a casserole dish and fry the onion for 10 mins until beginning to soften. Add the garlic, ground coriander and coriander stalks, and cook for 1 min. Stir though the tomatoes, stock and chipotle and bring to a simmer. Cook, covered, over a low heat for 20 mins, stirring occasionally.

STEP 2

Meanwhile, bring a pan of water to the boil and cook the corn for 4 mins. Drain and leave to cool a little. Cut the kernels off the cob with a sharp knife. Heat a non-stick frying pan over a high heat. Add the corn and fry for 5-7 mins or until charred, stirring now and again.

Creamy pumpkin & lentil soup

<u>Ingredients</u>

1 tbsp olive oil, plus 1 tsp

2 onions, chopped

2 garlic cloves, chopped

approx 800g chopped pumpkin flesh, plus the seeds

100g split red lentil

½ small pack thyme, leaves picked, plus extra to serve

1l hot vegetable stock

pinch of salt and sugar

50g crème fraîche, plus extra to serve

<u>Preparation</u>

STEP 1

Heat the oil in a large pan. Fry the onions until softened and starting to turn golden. Stir in the garlic, pumpkin flesh, lentils and thyme, then pour in the hot stock. Season, cover and simmer for 20-25 mins until the lentils and vegetables are tender.

STEP 2

Meanwhile, wash the pumpkin seeds. Remove any flesh still clinging to them, then dry them with kitchen paper. Heat the 1 tsp oil in a non-stick pan and fry the seeds until they start to jump and pop. Stir frequently, but cover the pan in between to keep them in it. When the seeds look nutty and toasted, add a sprinkling of salt and a pinch of sugar, and stir well.

Chorizo & chickpea soup

Ingredients

400g can chopped tomato

110g pack of chorizo sausage (unsliced)

140g wedge Savoy cabbage

sprinkling dried chilli flakes

410g can chickpea, drained and rinsed

1 chicken or vegetable stock cube

crusty bread or garlic bread, to serve

Preparation

STEP 1

Put a medium pan on the heat and tip in the tomatoes, followed by a can of water. While the tomatoes are heating, quickly chop the chorizo into chunky pieces (removing any skin) and shred the cabbage.

STEP 2

Pile the chorizo and cabbage into the pan with the chilli flakes and chickpeas, then crumble in the stock cube. Stir well, cover and leave to bubble over a high heat for 6 mins or until the cabbage is just tender. Ladle into bowls and eat with crusty or garlic bread.

White velvet soup with smoky almonds

<u>Ingredients</u>

2 tsp rapeseed oil

2 large garlic cloves, sliced

2 leeks, trimmed so they're mostly white in colour, washed well, then sliced (about 240g)

200g cauliflower, chopped

2 tsp vegetable bouillon powder

400g cannellini beans, rinsed

fresh nutmeg, for grating

100ml whole milk

25g whole almonds, chopped

½ tsp smoked paprika

2 x 25g slices rye bread, to serve

Preparation

STEP 1

Heat the oil in a large pan. Add the garlic, leeks and cauliflower and cook for about 5 mins, stirring frequently, until starting to soften (but not colouring).

STEP 2

Stir in the vegetable bouillon and beans, pour in 600ml boiling water and add a few generous gratings of the nutmeg. Cover and leave to simmer for 15 mins until the leeks and cauliflower are tender. Add the milk and blitz with a hand blender until smooth and creamy.

STEP 3

Put the almonds in a dry pan and cook very gently for 1 min, or until toasted, then remove from the heat. Scatter the paprika over the almonds and mix well. Ladle the soup into bowls, top with the spicy nuts and serve with the rye bread.

PART V

LIFESTYLE TIPS FOR SJÖGREN'S SYNDROME MANAGEMENT

Like any chronic condition, Sjögren's can take a toll on your emotional health and your body. To best manage:

Educate yourself: Learn as much as you can about the condition so you understand your options and know what to expect.

Join a support group: It can help get in touch with others who are going through the same thing. You can compare notes about symptoms and get ideas about what brings relief. The Sjögren's Syndrome Foundation can connect you with other. Or talk to your doctor about support groups in your area.

Family and friends, too, can be a great source of emotional support.

Take steps to care for your mental health: Be aware of what's burdening you, and work with a counselor or your support network to deal with these things. Keep in mind that your emotional state plays a role in the health of your body and your mind.

Request accommodations: If your condition interferes with your ability to do your job, consider asking for workplace changes like extra breaks or flexible hours.

www.ingramcontent.com/pod-product-compliance
Lightning Source LLC
Chambersburg PA
CBHW061035250726
48653CB00001B/98